Plain Talk for Patients

Plain Talk for Patients

Understanding Your Health in Clear, Simple Language

Sylvalene Alozie, DNP, MSN, BSN, APRN, FNP-C

First Edition — 2026 Printed in the United States of America

Copyright Page

Permissions & Licensing For permissions, bulk purchasing, clinic/organization licensing, educational distribution, or speaking inquiries, contact: Email: Metromed2026@gmail.com Website: Coming soon

Medical Disclaimer / Educational Use Statement

Important Notice (Please Read)

This book is for educational and informational purposes only. It does not provide medical advice, diagnosis, or treatment and is not a substitute for care from a licensed healthcare provider.

Healthcare decisions should always be made with your clinician, based on your medical history, symptoms, and test results. If you have questions about a test result, medication, new symptom, or treatment plan, contact your healthcare provider.

Do not ignore, delay, or stop medical care because of something you read in this book.

Emergency Warning: If you experience severe symptoms such as chest pain, trouble breathing, severe abdominal pain, signs of stroke (face drooping, arm weakness, speech difficulty), fainting, uncontrolled bleeding, or any symptoms that feel life-threatening, call 911 (or your local emergency number) or go to the nearest emergency department immediately.

The author and publisher are not responsible for outcomes related to how the information in this book is used. Your care team is the best source for advice specific to you.

Accessibility Note: If you need this information in another format or language, ask your clinic or healthcare organization about available patient education resources.

Dedication

For every patient who has ever read a medical report and felt uncertain before understanding.

May clear language bring you calm, compassionate conversations restore confidence, and every step of your healthcare journey remind you that you deserve clarity, respect, and peace of mind.

Reader Reassurance Page

A Note to You

If medical wording has ever made you feel anxious, confused, or overwhelmed, you are not alone. Many patients receive test results through online portals before a provider has the opportunity to explain what the language truly means. Seeing unfamiliar terms without context can make even routine findings feel frightening. Your reaction is human, valid, and understandable.

This book was created to help you feel steady again.

You do not need to become a medical expert to advocate for yourself. You simply need explanations that feel clear, respectful, and grounded in real understanding. Plain Talk for Patients™ exists to translate complex clinical language into calm, supportive guidance so you can approach your healthcare journey with greater

confidence.

As you read, keep these reminders close:

• An "abnormal" result is not automatically a diagnosis. • Imaging reports often describe what is seen — not the final meaning. • Words like "monitor," "follow-up," or "correlate clinically" are usually part of routine care, not a sign of crisis. • Your provider's interpretation — based on your full health story — is always the most important piece.

Take your time with this book. Pause when you need to. Highlight words that raise questions. Bring those questions into your healthcare conversations. Understanding grows step by step, and clarity often arrives when information is placed into the right context.

Most importantly, remember this: you deserve explanations that make sense. You deserve to feel heard, informed, and supported — not overwhelmed by medical language.

Plain Talk is here to help you replace fear with understanding, and uncertainty with calm.

How to Use This Book (Quick Start Guide)

Quick Start: How to Use Plain Talk for Patients

If you're reading this because your portal message made you anxious, start here:

Pause before you panic. Many results look scary without context.

Read for the "what," not the "why." Reports often describe what was seen—not the final meaning.

Look for next steps. Words like "follow-up," "repeat," or "correlate clinically" usually mean your provider will review and guide the plan.

Write down your questions. Use this book to translate terminology, then list what you want clarified.

Track your symptoms (if any). Symptoms matter. Tell your provider what you're feeling, when it started, and what makes it better or worse.

Avoid endless Googling. Online searches often show worst-case scenarios first. Use this book to stay grounded.

Bring this to your appointment. Highlight terms you want explained and ask your provider to put results in context.

Best way to read:

If you're overwhelmed, read one chapter at a time.

If you're reacting to labs, start with Chapter 2.

If you're reacting to imaging, start with Chapter 3.

Table of Contents

Introduction

If you have ever opened a patient portal and felt your heart race after reading a test result, you are not alone. Modern healthcare gives patients faster access to information than ever before, yet speed does not always come with clarity. Results are released instantly, medical terms appear without explanation, and many patients are left trying to interpret clinical language on their own.

Throughout my years in healthcare, I have learned that fear often begins long before a diagnosis is made. It starts when patients encounter words that sound serious but lack context. Terms like "abnormal," "lesion," or "follow-up recommended" may feel overwhelming, even when findings are mild or routine. This book was created to slow that moment down — to give you the understanding that often arrives too late.

Plain Talk for Patients is not meant to replace medical advice. Instead, it helps you understand the language surrounding your health so you can feel calmer, ask better questions, and walk into appointments with confidence. When patients understand what they are reading, they are less likely to imagine worst-case scenarios

and more likely to engage in meaningful conversations with their healthcare team.

Knowledge delivered with compassion can transform the healthcare experience. That is the purpose of Plain Talk — turning confusion into clarity and fear into understanding.

Chapter 1: Why Medical Language Feels Scary

Medical language is designed for accuracy, not comfort. Healthcare professionals rely on precise terminology to communicate efficiently, document findings clearly, and protect patient safety across teams. Every word used in a chart or report carries specific meaning within the clinical world. However, that same language can feel intimidating, cold, or even frightening when patients encounter it without explanation. Words like "abnormal," "lesion," "mass," or "inflammation" may sound severe, even though they are often neutral descriptions rather than diagnoses. To a clinician, these terms are simply part of a structured vocabulary. To a patient reading alone, they can feel like warning signs.

The challenge is not that medical language is wrong — it is that it was never designed to stand alone without context. Healthcare documentation prioritizes clarity between professionals, not emotional reassurance for readers. When patients access their records through portals, they are stepping into a conversation that was originally written for clinical communication. Without guidance, it is easy to misinterpret tone and meaning.

Many patients first encounter medical information during quiet, vulnerable moments — late at night, early in the morning, or between responsibilities. A notification appears, curiosity takes over, and within seconds unfamiliar words appear on a screen. Without a clinician present to explain the wording, the mind naturally begins to fill in gaps. Human nature leans toward protecting us from perceived threats, so it is common for people to imagine worst-case possibilities before hearing a professional interpretation.

Online searches often intensify this experience. While the internet provides access to information, it rarely offers balance. Severe conditions and rare diagnoses tend to appear more prominently in search results because they attract attention. A patient searching for the meaning of a single term may quickly encounter alarming explanations that do not reflect their individual situation. This can create a cycle of anxiety that grows long before a provider has reviewed the results or offered guidance.

Understanding the difference between description and diagnosis is one of the most powerful steps toward reducing fear. A radiology report may state that something "appears abnormal," but this does not mean a serious condition exists. It simply means that something looks different from what is typically expected and deserves closer review. Healthcare professionals use cautious wording to ensure accuracy, leaving room for clinical judgment once all information is considered. Observation always comes before interpretation.

For example, the word "lesion" often sounds alarming, yet it is simply a general term for an area that looks different from surrounding tissue. Many lesions are harmless and require only monitoring. Similarly, the word "mass" describes shape or structure, not severity. Even the term "inflammation" can represent temporary irritation rather than permanent damage. These words are tools clinicians use to communicate clearly — they are not conclusions about your health.

Recognizing this distinction can shift the emotional experience of reading medical information. Instead of viewing each unfamiliar term as a definitive statement, patients can begin to see reports as part of an ongoing process. Healthcare is rarely about a single result or isolated observation. Providers consider patterns, symptoms, medical history, and additional testing before forming a full picture. What appears concerning at first glance may ultimately be routine once placed into context.

Patients can protect their emotional well-being by creating a small pause between reading and reacting. Taking a breath, stepping away from the screen, or reminding yourself that results are only one piece of the puzzle can prevent the mind from moving too quickly toward fear. Writing down questions instead of searching endlessly online may also help shift focus from uncertainty to preparation for meaningful conversation.

Plain Talk encourages readers to approach medical wording with curiosity rather than alarm. Curiosity invites learning; fear often closes the door to understanding. When you view medical language as part of a structured system rather than a personal judgment, it becomes easier to remain grounded while waiting for clarification.

It is also helpful to remember that healthcare professionals understand how overwhelming medical terminology can feel. Providers, nurses, and clinical staff expect questions and welcome opportunities to explain results in a way that makes sense to you. Clear communication is not a burden — it is a vital part of safe and compassionate care.

Ultimately, interpretation always comes after observation. A report describes what was seen; your healthcare team determines what it means for you specifically. By allowing space for that process, you give yourself the opportunity to experience healthcare information with greater calm and confidence. Plain Talk exists to support that shift — transforming unfamiliar language into understanding, and helping you move from fear toward clarity.

Chapter 2: Understanding Lab Results in Plain Language

Lab results are one of the most common sources of confusion and anxiety for patients. A notification appears, numbers fill the screen, and suddenly familiar colors — red arrows, bold highlights, or words like "high" and "low" — can make even minor variations feel urgent. Many patients assume that anything outside the reference range means something is wrong.

In reality, healthcare providers rarely interpret lab results based on a single number alone. Instead, they look at patterns over time, symptoms, medications, and your overall health story.

Laboratory testing is designed to gather information, not deliver final conclusions. Each result represents a small piece of a much larger picture. When viewed without context, numbers may feel overwhelming, but when interpreted alongside clinical knowledge, they become helpful tools that guide decision-making rather than sources of fear.

Why Lab Numbers Can Feel Alarming

Reference ranges are often misunderstood. These ranges are created using averages from large groups of people, which means they represent typical values — not perfect definitions of health. Some individuals naturally fall slightly above or below these ranges and remain completely healthy. Seeing a result marked in red may simply indicate that your number sits just outside a statistical boundary, not that a serious condition exists.

Additionally, many everyday factors influence lab results. Hydration, sleep, recent meals, stress, medications, or even the time of day can cause temporary changes. Providers consider whether a variation is consistent over time or whether it may be a one-time shift before deciding if further action is necessary.

Understanding that lab results are part of a process — rather than a final judgment — can change how patients experience them. Instead of viewing each number as a verdict, it helps to see labs as information that helps your healthcare team understand your body more clearly.

Complete Blood Count (CBC): A Snapshot of Blood Health

A Complete Blood Count evaluates red blood cells, white blood cells, and platelets. These components help providers understand oxygen delivery, immune response, and clotting ability. Patients often worry when they see slight changes in hemoglobin, hematocrit, or white blood cell count, yet many variations are temporary.

Dehydration, minor infections, inflammation, or even recent physical activity can influence CBC values. A slightly elevated white blood cell count, for example, does not always indicate serious infection — it may simply reflect your body responding to stress or healing. Providers look at trends across multiple tests rather than reacting to a single result in isolation.

Learning to view CBC results as a snapshot rather than a definitive answer can reduce unnecessary worry and help patients focus on the broader context of their health.

Comprehensive Metabolic Panel (CMP): Looking at the Whole System

The Comprehensive Metabolic Panel provides insight into several areas at once, including kidney function, liver enzymes, electrolyte balance, and blood sugar levels. Because it evaluates multiple systems simultaneously, providers often focus on how numbers relate to one another rather than examining each result individually.

For example, slightly elevated liver enzymes may prompt providers to review medications, lifestyle factors, or recent illnesses before assuming a serious condition. Electrolyte levels may change temporarily with hydration or diet. Blood sugar levels can vary based on recent meals or stress levels.

Understanding that CMP results are interpreted as a group can help patients avoid becoming overly focused on one number. Providers use these patterns to guide conversations, recommend monitoring, or suggest lifestyle adjustments — not to deliver immediate conclusions without context.

Hemoglobin A1c: A Long-Term Perspective

Hemoglobin A1c provides a long-term view of blood sugar trends over several months. Unlike a single glucose reading, which captures a moment in time, A1c reflects patterns that develop gradually. Patients sometimes feel discouraged when they notice a slight increase, yet providers often interpret this result within the larger framework of lifestyle changes, medication adjustments, and individual goals.

Small shifts in A1c do not always require dramatic changes. Instead, they may serve as opportunities for conversation about nutrition, activity levels, or stress management. Understanding that A1c represents progress over time — rather than a single moment — helps patients approach the result with patience and perspective.

Cholesterol Panels: Understanding Risk, Not Judgment

Cholesterol panels measure different types of fats in the blood, including LDL, HDL, and triglycerides. These numbers help providers evaluate long-term heart health risk rather than immediate illness. Patients sometimes feel alarmed when they see cholesterol values outside the recommended range, but these numbers are tools for prevention and planning — not instant diagnoses.

Providers consider factors such as age, family history, blood pressure, and lifestyle habits when interpreting cholesterol results. Two individuals with similar numbers may receive different recommendations based on their overall health picture. Understanding this individualized approach can help patients view cholesterol panels as part of an ongoing conversation about wellness rather than a source of fear.

Seeing Lab Results Through a Broader Lens

One of the most important lessons in understanding lab results is recognizing that numbers rarely stand alone. Providers compare current values with past trends, evaluate symptoms, and consider your unique health history before deciding what any result truly means. A single abnormal value may simply signal the need for monitoring rather than immediate intervention.

When reviewing labs, it can be helpful to pause before reacting emotionally. Ask yourself: Is this a new pattern, or could it be a temporary change? Writing down questions for your provider instead of searching endlessly online can also reduce anxiety and help you feel more prepared for meaningful conversations.

Reference ranges are statistical averages — not strict boundaries between health and illness. Many healthy individuals fall slightly outside these ranges at times. Understanding that providers interpret labs within context allows patients to approach their results with greater calm and confidence.

Plain Talk encourages readers to see lab results not as judgments, but as tools for understanding the body's story. When numbers are placed into perspective, they become less intimidating and more empowering — guiding conversations that support long-term health and informed decision-making.

Chapter 3: Imaging Reports Explained

Imaging reports are often filled with technical language because radiologists must document findings with precision and clarity. Every word used in an imaging report serves a specific purpose within the medical system. Terms such as "lesion," "mass," "density," or "thickening" are not designed to frighten patients — they are descriptive tools that help clinicians communicate what was observed on a scan. These words describe appearance, shape, or structure. They do not automatically define a diagnosis or predict an outcome.

For many patients, however, imaging reports can feel overwhelming. Reading unfamiliar medical terminology without explanation may create the impression that something serious has been discovered. The truth is that radiology language is intentionally cautious. Radiologists describe exactly what they see while leaving room for providers to interpret the findings within the context of the patient's full health story.

Why Imaging Language Sounds More Serious Than It Is

Radiologists are trained to document observations carefully. Unlike casual conversation, medical imaging reports must remain precise and neutral. Words like “abnormal” or “suspicious” may sound alarming to someone outside healthcare, yet these terms often mean only that an area looks different from what is typically expected.

For example, a “lesion” simply refers to an area that appears distinct from surrounding tissue. It might represent a harmless cyst, scar tissue from a past injury, or even a normal anatomical variation. The word “mass” describes a shape or structure seen on imaging — not whether it is benign or malignant. Similarly, “thickening” may indicate inflammation, healing, or a temporary change rather than a serious condition.

Radiologists avoid making assumptions beyond what the images show. Their role is to describe, not to diagnose in isolation. This careful wording protects patients by ensuring that conclusions are based on the full clinical picture rather than a single snapshot.

Understanding Phrases That Often Cause Anxiety

Certain phrases appear frequently in imaging reports and can easily be misunderstood.

“Cannot rule out” does not mean something is present. It means the radiologist is leaving space for additional clinical evaluation.

“Recommend correlation” suggests that findings should be interpreted alongside symptoms or other tests.

"Clinical follow-up advised" often reflects caution rather than urgency.

These phrases are part of responsible medical documentation. They allow healthcare teams to consider multiple possibilities while maintaining accuracy. When patients understand that this language is protective rather than predictive, imaging reports often feel less intimidating.

Why Radiologists May Not Have the Full Story

Radiologists interpret images based primarily on visual information. While they may receive brief clinical notes, they do not always have access to every detail about a patient's symptoms, history, or recent changes. This is why your primary provider plays such an important role after imaging is completed.

Your provider reviews imaging results alongside lab values, physical exam findings, and your personal medical history. A finding that appears concerning on a report may ultimately be routine once viewed within this broader context. Conversely, a subtle change may become meaningful when combined with specific symptoms. Imaging is one piece of a much larger conversation about your health.

Understanding this collaborative process can help patients avoid placing too much weight on a single report. Imaging is a tool — not a final answer.

The Emotional Experience of Reading Imaging Reports

Many patients describe feeling anxious or unsettled when reading imaging results before speaking with their provider. This reaction is completely normal. The human mind naturally seeks certainty, and medical wording often feels ambiguous or technical.

One helpful approach is to shift focus from individual words to the overall purpose of the report. Instead of asking, "What does this term mean for my future?" consider asking, "What information does this give my healthcare team?" This small change in perspective can reduce emotional intensity and encourage a more balanced understanding.

It can also help to remember that imaging technology is incredibly sensitive. Modern scans detect small details that may never cause symptoms or require treatment. Not every finding represents a problem — many simply reflect the body's natural variations.

Seeing Imaging as Part of a Larger Puzzle

Healthcare decisions are rarely made based on imaging alone. Providers consider patterns over time, previous studies, symptoms, and risk factors before deciding whether follow-up is needed. Sometimes the most appropriate plan is simply monitoring — a strategy that allows clinicians to observe changes gradually rather than rushing toward intervention.

Plain Talk encourages readers to view imaging reports as pieces of a larger puzzle rather than standalone conclusions. Just as a single photograph cannot tell the entire story of a person's life, a single scan cannot define your health journey. It provides valuable information, but interpretation always comes through collaboration between you and your healthcare team.

Approaching Imaging Reports with Confidence

When reading imaging results, try to pause before interpreting unfamiliar terms as definitive answers.

Writing down questions for your provider can help transform uncertainty into productive conversation. Consider asking:

What does this finding usually represent?

Is this something that requires immediate attention or routine monitoring?

How does this result fit with my symptoms and history?

These questions shift the focus from fear toward understanding.

Understanding the cautious nature of imaging language allows patients to approach reports with greater perspective. Rather than focusing on individual words, consider imaging as one step in a thoughtful, structured process designed to support safe and informed care decisions.

Plain Talk reminds readers that imaging reports are not verdicts — they are tools that guide conversation, clarify next steps, and help healthcare teams provide the most appropriate care. When viewed through this lens, imaging language becomes less intimidating and more empowering, helping patients move forward with clarity rather than uncertainty.

Chapter 4: Common Gastrointestinal Terms Made Simple

Digestive health concerns are extremely common, yet many gastrointestinal (GI) terms sound intimidating when patients hear them for the first time. Words like “reflux,” “gastritis,” “diverticulosis,” or “inflammation” may feel heavy or unfamiliar, even though these conditions are often manageable and widely experienced. Much of the anxiety surrounding GI terminology comes not from the condition itself, but from the way the language is presented. When patients understand what these words truly mean — and what they do not mean — the experience often shifts from fear to confidence.

The digestive system is complex, and providers use specific terms to describe how different parts of the gastrointestinal tract function. These terms help clinicians communicate clearly, but they can sound more serious than intended when heard outside of a medical setting. Plain Talk focuses on translating this language into explanations that feel understandable and grounded in real-life experience.

Understanding Reflux in Plain Language

Reflux occurs when stomach acid moves upward into the esophagus, sometimes causing burning in the chest or throat, a sour taste, or frequent throat clearing. Many people associate reflux with severe illness, yet it is one of the most common digestive concerns worldwide. Factors such as certain foods, meal timing, stress, or body position can influence symptoms.

While reflux can be uncomfortable, it is often manageable through lifestyle adjustments and medication when needed. Providers may recommend changes such as avoiding late-night meals, reducing acidic foods, or elevating the head during sleep. Understanding that reflux exists on a spectrum — from occasional symptoms to chronic conditions — helps patients approach treatment with balance rather than fear.

Gastritis: Understanding Irritation Versus Damage

The word "gastritis" simply refers to inflammation or irritation of the stomach lining. Patients sometimes imagine severe injury when they hear this term, yet gastritis can develop from temporary triggers such as medications, stress, certain foods, or infections. In many cases, the stomach lining heals once these triggers are addressed.

Providers may recommend medications that reduce acid production or protect the stomach while it recovers. Lifestyle adjustments, such as avoiding irritating foods or limiting alcohol intake, may also play a role. Understanding that gastritis often represents a reversible process can help patients feel less overwhelmed when they encounter the diagnosis.

Diverticulosis: A Common Finding, Not a Crisis

Diverticulosis describes small pouches that form in the colon over time. This is a very common finding, especially as people age, and many individuals live with diverticulosis without ever experiencing symptoms. The word itself may sound alarming, but it does not automatically indicate illness or danger.

Providers often emphasize hydration, balanced nutrition, and fiber intake as part of maintaining colon health. Occasionally, these pouches may become irritated, leading to a condition called diverticulitis, which requires medical attention. However, the presence of diverticulosis alone is not a sign of severe disease. Learning the difference between these terms helps patients avoid unnecessary worry.

Why GI Procedures Are Often Preventative

Hearing that an endoscopy or colonoscopy is recommended can cause immediate anxiety for many patients. These procedures are frequently misunderstood as signals of serious illness, when in reality they are often preventative tools designed to protect long-term health.

An endoscopy allows providers to examine the esophagus and stomach to better understand symptoms such as reflux or discomfort. A colonoscopy helps evaluate the colon and screen for changes that may develop slowly over time. These tests are valuable because they allow providers to detect issues early — often before symptoms become severe.

Understanding the purpose behind these procedures can change how patients view them. Rather than seeing them as signs of something wrong, they can be viewed as proactive steps toward maintaining wellness.

The Role of Language in Shaping Fear

Many GI terms sound unfamiliar because they originate from medical terminology rather than everyday language. Words like "esophagitis," "polyps," or "biopsy" may feel intimidating simply because they are new. When these terms are explained clearly, patients often realize that they describe routine processes within digestive care.

Plain Talk encourages readers to ask for explanations whenever terminology feels confusing. Providers expect questions and understand that clear communication is essential for patient comfort. By seeking clarification, patients move from feeling overwhelmed to feeling informed and engaged.

Lifestyle, Education, and Collaboration

One of the most empowering aspects of GI health is that many digestive conditions improve with education and lifestyle adjustments. Small changes — such as modifying diet, managing stress, staying hydrated, or adjusting meal timing — can make a meaningful difference in symptoms. Medication may be helpful in certain situations, but understanding the role of daily habits often gives patients a sense of control over their health journey.

Collaboration between patients and providers plays a central role in managing GI conditions. When patients understand terminology and feel comfortable discussing symptoms openly, providers can tailor recommendations more effectively. Clear explanations create a foundation of trust, allowing patients to participate actively in decisions about their care.

Seeing GI Terminology Through a New Lens

Digestive health language may sound intimidating at first, but most GI terms simply describe processes happening within the body. Reflux reflects movement of acid, gastritis describes irritation, and diverticulosis refers to structural changes that often occur naturally over time. Understanding these terms in plain language helps patients see that many digestive conditions are manageable and common.

Plain Talk encourages readers to approach GI terminology with curiosity rather than fear. Knowledge transforms unfamiliar words into understandable concepts, allowing patients to feel calmer and more confident when discussing digestive health. When explanations are clear and compassionate, GI care becomes less about worrying over terminology and more about building a plan that supports long-term wellness.

Chapter 5: Liver Health in Plain Talk

Liver health can feel especially intimidating because the liver plays such a central role in keeping the body balanced. It helps process nutrients, filter substances from the bloodstream, regulate energy, and support countless metabolic functions. When patients hear that something involving the liver is "abnormal," it can immediately trigger worry. However, many liver-related findings are far more common — and often far less severe — than people initially assume.

One of the most frequent sources of anxiety comes from elevated liver enzymes. Patients often see numbers outside the reference range and fear that permanent damage has already occurred. In reality, liver enzymes are markers of irritation, not automatic proof of disease. Temporary factors such as medications, recent illness, alcohol intake, dehydration, or metabolic changes can influence these values. Providers look at trends over time rather than reacting to a single result in isolation.

Understanding Liver Enzymes Without Panic

Liver enzyme tests, including AST, ALT, and alkaline phosphatase, provide clues about how the liver is functioning. Slight elevations may reflect inflammation or stress on the liver rather than irreversible injury. Much like a fever signal that the body is responding to something, enzyme changes can indicate that the liver is reacting — not necessarily failing.

It is important to remember that laboratory values fluctuate. A mildly elevated result today may return to normal later once the underlying cause resolves. Providers often repeat tests or monitor levels before drawing conclusions. Understanding this process can help patients approach liver lab results with patience rather than fear.

What "Fatty Liver" Really Means

Terms such as "fatty liver" or "hepatic steatosis" have become increasingly common in imaging reports and clinic visits. These phrases describe the presence of extra fat within liver cells — a condition often linked to metabolic health, nutrition, or insulin resistance. While the wording may sound alarming, fatty liver exists on a spectrum, and many individuals experience improvement through gradual lifestyle adjustments.

Healthcare providers focus on sustainable changes rather than drastic measures. Balanced nutrition, physical activity, and management of conditions such as diabetes or high cholesterol may all support liver health over time. For many patients, understanding that fatty liver can improve helps shift the focus from fear to proactive action.

Monitoring Does Not Mean Decline

Another common misconception is that frequent monitoring indicates worsening health. In liver care, monitoring is often a sign of prevention. Providers track lab trends and imaging results to ensure that changes remain stable or improve over time. Follow-up testing allows healthcare teams to identify patterns early and adjust care plans thoughtfully.

Patients sometimes feel discouraged when they hear that repeat labs or imaging are recommended. However, monitoring is not a sign that something is wrong — it is a way of staying informed and protecting long-term health. When viewed through this lens, follow-up becomes a form of reassurance rather than a source of anxiety.

Seeing Liver Health as a Spectrum

One of the most helpful ways to understand liver health is to think of it as a continuum rather than a single diagnosis. Just as blood pressure or blood sugar can change gradually, liver function reflects many different influences over time. Lifestyle habits, genetics, medications, and underlying health conditions all play a role.

Providers consider trends across months or years, imaging findings, and individual risk factors before making recommendations. A single lab value rarely tells the full story. Understanding this broader perspective allows patients to focus on progress rather than perfection.

Balancing Information with Emotional Well-Being

Because the liver is such a vital organ, discussions about liver health can feel emotionally heavy. Patients may imagine worst-case scenarios when they see unfamiliar terminology or hear that results are being monitored. Plain Talk encourages readers to approach liver information with balance — recognizing that many findings are manageable and that improvement often happens gradually.

Taking time to ask questions can be empowering. Patients may consider asking their provider:

What do this liver numbers suggest over time, not just today?

Are these changes mild, moderate, or significant?

What steps can I take that make the biggest difference right now?

These conversations help transform uncertainty into actionable understanding.

Education as a Tool for Confidence

Education plays a powerful role in shaping how patients experience liver health. When terminology is explained clearly, words like "steatosis" or "elevated enzymes" begin to feel less intimidating. Patients who understand their results are more likely to engage in care plans and feel confident about their ability to influence their health journey.

Plain Talk emphasizes that liver health is not defined by one number or one report. It is shaped by ongoing collaboration between patients and healthcare teams, guided by information, compassion, and thoughtful decision-making.

Moving Forward with Perspective

Understanding liver health as a spectrum — rather than a fixed label — helps patients focus on proactive steps instead of fear. Providers look at trends, imaging, symptoms, and risk factors before making recommendations, and many individuals experience improvement through gradual, sustainable changes.

When patients see liver care as a process rather than a crisis, the language surrounding it becomes less overwhelming. Knowledge allows you to approach liver results with clarity, balance, and confidence, recognizing that monitoring and education are powerful tools for maintaining long-term wellness.

Chapter 6: Questions Patients Should Feel Comfortable Asking

Effective healthcare conversations begin with curiosity. Yet many patients hesitate to ask questions during appointments. Some worry about taking too much time, while others fear appearing uninformed or challenging their provider. In reality, thoughtful questions are one of the most powerful tools patients have. They help healthcare professionals understand what matters most to you, clarify expectations, and ensure that information is truly understood.

Healthcare visits can move quickly. Providers often balance time constraints, documentation, and clinical decision-making all at once. Because of this, important details may feel rushed unless patients feel comfortable speaking up. Asking questions does not slow care — it strengthens it. When patients share their concerns openly, providers can tailor explanations and recommendations in ways that feel more personal and meaningful.

Why Patients Sometimes Hold Back

Many people were raised to see healthcare professionals as authority figures who should not be interrupted. Others assume that if something were important, the provider would mention it without being asked. Some patients simply feel overwhelmed by unfamiliar terminology and are unsure where to begin.

These reactions are understandable, but silence can lead to confusion after the appointment ends. Patients may leave with unanswered questions, turn to internet searches for clarity, or feel uncertain about what steps to take next. Creating space for curiosity during the visit helps prevent this cycle and allows patients to leave with a stronger sense of understanding.

Questions That Create Clarity

Simple, direct questions can transform the experience of a healthcare visit. Consider asking:

What does this result mean in simple language? Providers may use technical terminology out of habit, but most are happy to rephrase information in everyday terms. This question invites clearer communication without requiring medical knowledge.

Is this urgent or routine follow-up? Understanding the level of urgency helps reduce anxiety and sets realistic expectations about timing. Many findings require monitoring rather than immediate action.

What changes, if any, should I make right now? Patients often leave appointments unsure whether lifestyle adjustments, medication changes, or further testing are needed. Clarifying next steps provides a sense of direction.

When should I expect to hear back about next steps? Knowing the timeline for results or follow-up appointments can ease uncertainty and prevent unnecessary worry while waiting.

These questions are not confrontational — they are collaborative. They help ensure that both patient and provider share the same understanding moving forward.

Preparing for Appointments with Confidence

Preparation can make a significant difference in how patients experience healthcare visits. Writing down questions ahead of time allows you to stay focused, especially if emotions run high during the appointment. Some patients find it helpful to keep a small notebook or use a notes app on their phone to track symptoms, concerns, or changes between visits.

Bringing a trusted friend or family member can also provide support, particularly during complex discussions. Another person may remember details that are easy to forget in the moment. Asking for written summaries or after-visit instructions can further improve understanding once you return home.

The Value of Writing Things Down

Healthcare conversations often involve a lot of information in a short amount of time. Writing down explanations during visits can help you recall details later and reduce the need to rely solely on memory. Patients sometimes feel hesitant to take notes, but most providers welcome this practice because it shows engagement and commitment to understanding.

If something remains unclear after the appointment, it is perfectly reasonable to reach out through a patient portal or follow-up call. Communication does not end when the visit concludes; it continues as part of an ongoing partnership.

Creating a True Partnership with Your Healthcare Team

Healthcare works best when patients and providers communicate openly. Providers bring clinical expertise, while patients bring personal experience — knowledge about their symptoms, lifestyle, and goals. When both perspectives come together, care becomes more personalized and effective.

Asking questions signals that you are invested in your health journey. It allows providers to adjust explanations, clarify misunderstandings, and ensure that recommendations align with your priorities. This shared decision-making process strengthens trust and helps patients feel more confident in the path forward.

Overcoming the Fear of "Asking Too Much"

One of the most common concerns patients express is the fear of asking too many questions. It is important to remember that healthcare providers expect curiosity. Questions help them understand whether information has been communicated clearly. If time is limited during a visit, providers may suggest scheduling a follow-up discussion — not because questions are unwelcome, but because they want to give thoughtful answers.

Patients who feel empowered to ask questions often report feeling calmer and more in control of their healthcare experience. Curiosity transforms appointments from passive conversations into active collaborations.

Moving Forward with Confidence

Preparing questions before appointments, writing down key points, and seeking clarification when needed all contribute to a more positive healthcare experience. Plain Talk encourages readers to see themselves as active participants in their care — individuals whose voices matter just as much as the medical information being discussed.

Remember that healthcare is not a one-sided process. Providers want patients to feel informed and supported. Asking questions creates opportunities for clearer communication, stronger relationships, and decisions that reflect both clinical expertise and personal understanding.

When curiosity replaces hesitation, healthcare conversations become more meaningful, more collaborative, and far less intimidating.

Chapter 7: Reducing Anxiety While Waiting for Results

Waiting for medical results can feel emotionally draining. Many patients describe checking their patient portal repeatedly throughout the day, replaying conversations in their mind, or imagining worst-case scenarios while they wait for answers. Even when daily life continues — work responsibilities, family obligations, or social commitments — uncertainty can quietly sit in the background, making it difficult to feel fully present.

These reactions are completely normal. The human brain naturally seeks certainty, especially when health is involved. When answers feel just out of reach, the mind may try to fill the silence with assumptions. Understanding that this response is a natural part of being human can help reduce self-judgment during waiting periods.

Why Waiting Feels So Difficult

Healthcare timelines often move differently from everyday expectations. Patients may expect immediate answers after testing, yet many results require careful review. Providers compare current findings with previous tests, consult with specialists, and evaluate information within the context of your personal health history. While this thoughtful process protects patient safety, it can feel frustrating when you are waiting for clarity.

Digital portals have changed how patients experience this time. Notifications can arrive quickly, but interpretation may take longer. Seeing partial information without explanation can intensify anxiety. It is important to remember that delays often reflect careful decision-making rather than neglect or urgency.

Focusing on What You Can Control

One of the most effective ways to manage anxiety during waiting periods is to focus on actions that support your well-being. While you may not control when results are finalized, you can influence how you care for yourself in the meantime.

Limiting excessive internet searches is a powerful first step. Online information can be helpful, but it often presents extreme scenarios that do not apply to most people. Constant searching may increase worry rather than provide reassurance. Choosing reliable sources — or waiting for guidance from your healthcare provider — can protect your emotional balance.

Maintaining routines can also create stability. Regular movement, balanced meals, hydration, and consistent sleep patterns help regulate stress responses within the body. These simple actions remind you that life continues beyond the uncertainty of waiting.

The Value of Connection and Support

Talking with trusted friends or family members can provide comfort during times of uncertainty. Sharing your thoughts aloud may help you process emotions and feel less alone. Some patients find reassurance in connecting with others who have experienced similar health concerns, while others prefer quiet reflection. There is no single right way to navigate waiting — only what feels supportive for you.

Writing down concerns can also be helpful. Instead of allowing worries to circulate endlessly in your mind, placing them on paper turns them into questions that can be addressed later. When results arrive, you will already have a starting point for conversation with your provider.

Understanding the Medical Review Process

Many patients assume that results should be interpreted immediately, yet healthcare decisions often involve multiple steps. A lab value may need confirmation, an imaging study may require comparison with previous scans, or a specialist may review findings before recommendations are made. These layers of review exist to ensure accuracy and protect patient safety.

Recognizing that thoughtful review takes time can help shift the meaning of waiting. Rather than viewing delays as signs of danger, they can be seen as evidence that your healthcare team is working carefully behind the scenes. Patience during this process allows providers to offer guidance that reflects the full picture rather than a rushed interpretation.

Creating Emotional Space During Uncertainty

During waiting periods, it can be helpful to create small moments of emotional distance from the situation. This does not mean ignoring your health — it means allowing yourself permission to rest from constant worry. Engaging in hobbies, spending time outdoors, or practicing simple breathing exercises can help calm the nervous system.

Some patients find comfort in setting boundaries around when they check their portal. Instead of refreshing repeatedly throughout the day, choosing specific times to review updates may reduce emotional fatigue. Small changes in how you engage with information can make a meaningful difference in how waiting feels.

Transforming Waiting into Preparation

Waiting does not have to be a passive experience. It can become a time of preparation. Consider reflecting on what matters most to you: your goals, concerns, or preferences related to your health. Writing down these thoughts allows you to enter follow-up conversations with clarity and confidence.

Preparing questions ahead of time also helps shift focus away from fear and anxiety. Instead of wondering "What if something is wrong?" you might ask, "What information will help me feel prepared for the next step?" This mindset turns uncertainty into an opportunity for growth and understanding.

Moving Through Waiting with Compassion

Patience during the medical review process allows healthcare professionals to provide thoughtful, individualized guidance. While waiting can feel uncomfortable, it is often a sign that your care is being approached with care and precision.

Plain Talk encourages readers to view waiting not as a void filled with fear, but as a space for reflection, self-care, and preparation. Understanding that many results require comparison, consultation, and careful interpretation can help transform uncertainty into trust.

When you approach waiting with compassion toward yourself, you create room for calm even before answers arrive. Healthcare journeys are rarely defined by a single moment — they unfold over time, guided by information, collaboration, and thoughtful care.

Chapter 8: Partnering With Your Healthcare Team

Healthcare works best when patients and providers move forward together. While medical professionals bring clinical knowledge and experience, patients bring something equally important — personal insight into their own bodies, lifestyles, and goals. When these perspectives come together through open communication, healthcare becomes more collaborative, more supportive, and often more effective.

Many people grow up believing that healthcare is something done to them rather than with them. Appointments may feel rushed, medical language may sound unfamiliar, and it can be easy to assume that decisions are made solely by clinicians. In reality, modern healthcare thrives on partnership. Nurses, medical assistants, specialists, and primary providers each contribute to helping you understand your health journey, but your voice remains a central part of that process.

Understanding the Roles Within Your Care Team

A healthcare team often includes several professionals working behind the scenes. Nurses help translate medical information, provide education, and monitor changes over time. Medical assistants support communication and coordination, helping ensure that appointments and follow-up plans run smoothly. Providers — such as physicians, nurse practitioners, or physician assistants — evaluate findings, make diagnoses, and guide treatment decisions.

Recognizing that each person plays a different role can make interactions feel less overwhelming. When patients understand who to turn to for specific questions or concerns, communication becomes more efficient and supportive. The healthcare system may feel complex at times, but its purpose is to provide layers of care that work together for your benefit.

The Power of Open and Respectful Communication

Partnership begins with communication that feels open, respectful, and honest. Patients sometimes hesitate to share concerns because they worry about being judged or misunderstood. Yet providers rely on honest feedback to make informed decisions. Describing symptoms clearly, sharing lifestyle challenges, or expressing fears allows your healthcare team to tailor recommendations that truly fit your life.

Respect flows in both directions. Providers aim to offer expertise and guidance, while patients bring lived experience and personal values to every conversation. When both voices are welcomed, understanding deepens and trust grows naturally. Over time, this trust can transform healthcare visits from stressful obligations into meaningful opportunities for connection, reassurance, and healing. In these moments, patients feel seen, heard, and supported — not just treated. Clear, compassionate communication helps reduce fear and builds confidence in the care plan. When patients understand what's happening and why, they are more empowered to participate in decisions about their health.

Why Feeling Informed Changes Outcomes

Patients who feel informed are often more confident in following treatment plans and recognizing changes early. Understanding why a medication is prescribed or why a test is recommended makes it easier to stay engaged in the process. Education does not just provide knowledge — it creates a sense of ownership over your health journey.

When patients feel comfortable asking questions and seeking clarification, misunderstandings decrease. Clear communication helps prevent confusion after appointments and reduces the need for repeated explanations later. Providers appreciate patients who actively participate because it strengthens collaboration and improves long-term outcomes.

Finding Your Voice in Healthcare Conversations

Building a partnership with your healthcare team means recognizing that your voice matters. You have the right to ask questions, request clarification, and express preferences about your care. Speaking up does not mean challenging expertise — it means contributing to a shared understanding.

Some patients find it helpful to prepare for appointments by writing down concerns or goals beforehand. Others prefer to reflect after visits and send follow-up questions through patient portals. There is no single way to participate; what matters most is feeling empowered to communicate openly.

It is also important to remember that healthcare decisions are rarely one-size-fits-all. Two patients with similar conditions may choose different approaches based on their values or circumstances. A strong partnership allows space for these differences, ensuring that care plans feel realistic and supportive.

Navigating Challenges with Compassion

Partnership does not mean that every interaction will feel easy. There may be moments when information feels overwhelming or when emotions run high. During these times, patience — both with yourself and with your healthcare team — can help maintain trust. If something feels unclear, it is always appropriate to ask for further explanation or to request additional time to process information.

Healthcare professionals understand that medical journeys can be emotional. They want patients to feel supported, not rushed. When conversations remain respectful and collaborative, even difficult topics can become opportunities for growth and understanding.

Seeing Yourself as an Active Participant

Plain Talk encourages readers to move away from the idea of being passive recipients of care. Instead, consider yourself an active participant — someone who brings insight, curiosity, and personal experience to the healthcare relationship. Your questions, observations, and feedback all contribute to the quality of your care.

Active participation does not require medical expertise. It simply involves staying engaged, asking for clarity when needed, and recognizing that your perspective is valuable. When patients feel seen and heard, healthcare becomes more human and less intimidating.

Moving Forward Together

Partnership with your healthcare team is built over time through shared experiences and honest communication. Each appointment, question, and conversation strengthens the connection between you and the people supporting your health. When communication feels open and respectful, trust grows — and with trust comes a greater sense of confidence in the journey ahead.

Plain Talk reminds readers that you deserve clarity, compassion, and understanding at every step of your healthcare experience. By embracing your role as a partner in care, you help create a space where knowledge and empathy meet — a space where healing is not only possible, but collaborative.

Conclusion

Medical language should never leave you feeling powerless. Yet for many patients, the experience of reading test results or hearing unfamiliar terminology can feel isolating and overwhelming. Behind every report, lab value, or imaging study is a team of professionals working carefully to understand your health in its full context. When explanations are clear and compassionate, anxiety begins to fade, and a sense of confidence can take its place.

Throughout this book, you have explored how words like "abnormal," "follow-up," "monitoring," or "inflammation" are often misunderstood outside the clinical setting. These terms are not final judgments about your health — they are part of a thoughtful process designed to gather information, guide decisions, and protect your well-being. Learning to view medical language through this lens allows you to approach healthcare conversations with a calmer and more informed perspective.

Plain Talk was created to transform complicated terminology into conversations that feel human and approachable. Healthcare does not have to feel distant or confusing. When information is explained in ways that respect both accuracy and emotion, patients begin to see their health journey differently. Instead of reacting to unfamiliar words with fear, you can approach them with curiosity — asking questions, seeking clarity, and trusting the process behind the language.

It is important to remember that your health is never defined by a single number, test result, or report. Providers consider patterns over time, personal history, lifestyle factors, and your own experiences when making decisions. Healthcare is rarely a straight line; it is a process that evolves through understanding, partnership, and communication. Recognizing this can help shift the focus away from momentary worry and toward long-term perspective.

Your role in this process matters. When patients feel informed, they become active participants rather than passive observers. Asking questions, seeking explanation, and sharing concerns openly strengthens the relationship between you and your healthcare team. Partnership does not mean having all the answers — it means feeling comfortable enough to ask for them.

There may still be moments when uncertainty feels heavy. Waiting for results, hearing new terminology, or navigating changes in health can bring understandable emotions. During those times, returning to the principles of Plain Talk can help ground you: pause before assuming the worst, look at the broader context, and allow space for thoughtful interpretation. Clarity often arrives when information is placed within the larger story of your health.

Knowledge delivered in plain language has the power to replace fear with understanding. It creates space for hope, resilience, and confidence — not because uncertainty disappears, but because you gain the tools to navigate it. Healthcare becomes less about decoding complex words and more about building meaningful conversations that support your well-being.

As you move forward, remember that your healthcare journey is shaped by collaboration and compassion. You deserve explanations that make sense, conversations that feel respectful, and care that recognizes you as a whole person — not just a diagnosis or a number on a page. When language becomes clear, the path ahead often feels less intimidating and more manageable.

That is the heart of Plain Talk: helping you move through healthcare with clarity, confidence, and hope. By understanding the language around your health, you take an important step toward feeling empowered in every conversation, every decision, and every stage of your journey.

About the Author

Sylvalene Alozie, DNP, MSN, BSN, APRN, FNP-C is a board-certified Family Nurse Practitioner devoted to patient education, preventive care, and advancing health literacy. She believes healthcare conversations should feel clear, respectful, and reassuring — never overwhelming or confusing.

Through the Plain Talk for Patients™ approach, she transforms complex medical language into simple, compassionate guidance that helps readers better understand their health and feel more confident during medical visits. Her work focuses on building trust, reducing fear, and empowering individuals to take an active role in their care.

Her mission is simple: to replace uncertainty with clarity and help every patient feel informed, supported, and heard.

www.ingramcontent.com/pod-product-compliance
Lightning Source LLC
LaVergne TN
LVHW090336210926
848480LV00004B/1429